LAVENDER

MARIAN KIM

ISBN: 1508664463

ISBN-13: 978-1508664468

CONTENTS

1

PROPERTIES

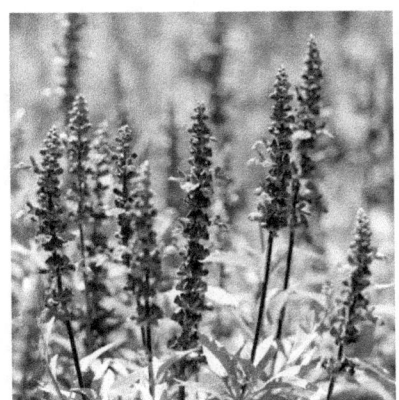

Scientific name: Lavandula angustifolia

Other names: Common lavender, English lavender and true lavender

Properties

Analgesic (pain relieving) properties

Anti-inflammatory properties

Antiseptic (antibacterial, antiviral, antifungal) properties

Emmenagogue (ability to stimulate blood flow in the pelvic area) properties

Immune system boosting properties

Mentally calming properties

Skin regenerating properties

Sebum (oil) balancing production

Sedative (sleep inducing) properties

2

USES

Alopecia areata treatment

Lavender stimulates hair growth and it is used for thinning hair and hair loss conditions. Lavender essential oil is used for alopecia areata when it is combined with thyme, rosemary and cedarwood essential oils.

Depression treatment

Lavender tincture is used for managing depression. Studies have shown that it is almost as effective as the prescription medication imipramine (Tofranil).

Insomnia treatment

Lavender has sedative or sleep inducing properties which are useful for treating insomnia (sleeplessness).

Studies have shown that the oil can assist with mild insomnia when inhaled from a vaporizer.

Migraine treatment

Lavender has analgesic (pain relieving) properties and is thus used for migraine headaches. Some studies suggest that massaging a few drops on the upper lip in order to inhale the lavender aroma can reduce the pain and nausea associated with migraines and possibly prevent it from spreading. Lavender is also used for toothaches.

Cuts, bruises and burns

Lavender has antiseptic (antibacterial, antiviral) properties and cell regenerating properties which help the skin heal faster and with less scarring. It is therefore used for minor cuts, bruises, burns and sunburns. It is also used for insect bites. Lavender infused oils, salves and poultices can be used for this purpose.

Acne treatment

Lavender is used for acne since it balances sebum (oil) production and it also has antiseptic (antibacterial) properties.

Athlete's foot treatment

Lavender has antifungal properties and is used for treating athlete's foot, ringworm and other fungal infections.

Eczema and psoriasis treatment

Lavender has anti-inflammatory properties and it is thus used for eczema and psoriasis. It is also used to manage psoriasis prone scalps. Lavender infused oils and salves can be used for this purpose.

Mature skin management

Lavender is used to manage mature and prematurely aging skin.

Sensitive skin management

Lavender is used to manage sensitive skin.

Dry skin management

Lavender balances sebum (oil) production and is therefore useful for managing dry skin types. Lavender infused oils and salves can be used for this purpose.

Repelling insects

Lavender has insect repellant properties and is used to repel mosquitoes and other insects.

Lice treatment

Lavender is used to treat lice.

Itchy scalp management

Lavender soothes inflamed and itchy scalps.

Dandruff treatment

Lavender balances scalp sebum (oil) production and is used to help manage dandruff. It is also used to manage dry hair.

Stress management

Lavender has scientifically proven mentally relaxing properties and it is used for stress management. It is also used for managing stress related symptoms like indigestion, nervous exhaustion and tension headaches.

Anxiety management

Lavender has calming effects and it is used to relieve anxiety. It is also used for restlessness and nervousness

Anger management

Lavender is used for anger management.

Urinary tract infections (UTI) treatment

Lavender has antiseptic properties and immune system boosting properties and is thus used for urinary tract infections (UTI).

Coughs and flu symptom management

Lavender has antiseptic properties and immune system boosting properties and is thus used for colds, coughs and the flu.

Arthritis treatment

Lavender has analgesic (pain relieving) properties and is thus used for arthritis, joint pains and backaches. It is also used for other painful conditions like muscle aches, spasms, sprains and neuralgia (nerve pain). Lavender infused oils or lavender salves can be used for this purpose.

PMS management

Lavender has emmenagogue properties or the ability to stimulate blood flow in the pelvic area and thus it is used for premenstrual tension (PMS).

Dysmenorrhea management

Lavender has analgesic (pain relieving) properties and is thus used for dysmenorrhea (painful periods.

Assisting delivery

Lavender has emmenagogue properties or the ability to stimulate blood flow in the pelvic area and thus it is used for assisting in child birth.

Digestive disorders

Lavender is used for digestive disorders like anorexia (loss of appetite), nausea, vomiting, colic, flatulence (intestinal gas) and upset stomachs.

* * * * *

3

SAFETY PRECAUTIONS

1. Do not use/avoid lavender if you are allergic to it.

2. Do not use /avoid lavender in pregnancy.

3. Do not use/avoid lavender if you are breastfeeding.

4. Do not use /avoid lavender on young children as it may cause premature breast development in boys and girls.

5. Do not use /avoid lavender if you have low blood pressure since you may feel drowsy after using it.

6. Do not use /avoid lavender if scheduled to have surgery within 2 weeks as it can slow the nervous system when combined with anesthetics.

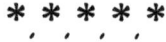

4

DRUG INTERACTIONS

1. Do not use/ avoid lavender herbal remedies if you are taking barbiturates like phenobarbital (Donnatal), amobarbital (Amytal), pentobarbital (Luminal) and secobarbital (Seconal) since you may develop excessive sleepiness.

2. Do not use/avoid lavender if you are taking sedatives or medications to help you sleep like zolpidem (Ambien) since you might develop excessive drowsiness.

3. Do not use/avoid lavender if you are taking anti-anxiety medications like diazepam and lorazepam (Ativan) to avoid developing excessive sleepiness.

4. Do not use/avoid lavender if you are taking narcotic pain relieving medications like morphine and oxycodone.

5. Do not use/avoid lavender if you are taking chloral hydrate since both medication cause drowsiness.

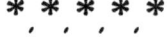

5

COOKING TIPS

Flavor

Sweet and floral

Goes well with

Sweet dishes like fruit pies, puddings, cakes, chocolate and jams. It is also used in breads and drinks like lemonade as well as ice cream.

Can be substituted with

Rosemary, sage, thyme

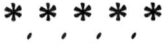

6

HERBAL RECIPES

Lavender Tea

Equipment

Tea pot or kettle

***

Ingredients

1 teaspoon of crushed lavender

1 cup of boiling water

Honey to taste (optional)

***

Instructions

1. Put the lavender in a tea pot or kettle, add the boiling water and let it steep while covered for 10 -15 minutes.

2. Add honey (if using) to suit your taste before drinking.

*****

Lavender Infusion

Equipment

Glass jar with tight fitting lid

***

Ingredients

1 teaspoon dried lavender flowers or 3 teaspoons fresh lavender

1 cup boiling water

***

Instructions

1. Place the lavender in the glass jar and add the boiling water.

2. Close the lid and let the mixture steep for 4 hours to 14 hours (overnight).

3. Strain the lavender and the infusion is ready for use.

4. Store the infusion in the refrigerator to lengthen its life.

*****

Lavender Compress

Equipment

Large bowl

Clean cloth or cotton balls

***

Ingredients

3 cups lavender infusion (see previous recipe)

***

Instructions

1. Pour the lavender infusion in the bowl.

2. Dip a clean cotton cloth in the infusion and squeeze out the excess fluid while making sure that you do not burn yourself.

3. Apply the lavender compress to the affected body part.

***

Tips

1. Lavender compresses are applied to the forehead to relieve headaches. If they are tension headaches, the compress can be applied to the base of the neck.

*****

Lavender Tincture

Equipment

Glass jar with tight fitting lid

Dark tincture bottles

Cheesecloth

***

Ingredients

7 oz (200 gm) of dried lavender or 14 oz (400 gm) of fresh lavender

30 oz (1 liter) of 80-100 proof vodka

***

Instructions

1. Fill 1/3 of the glass jar with the chopped lavender.

2. Add the vodka to completely fill the jar to the top.

3. Seal the jar and label it with the date of preparation and name of herb used.

4. Store the glass jar in a dark place for 6 weeks ensuring that you shake them weekly.

5. After 6 weeks strain out the lavender with a cheesecloth and pour the tincture into dark tincture bottles.

6. Label the tincture bottles with the date and name of herb used.

7. Store your herbal tinctures away from light and heat.

*****

Lavender Syrup

Equipment

Saucepan

Jar with airtight lid

***

Ingredients

1 quart (1000 ml) filtered water

1 cup lavender

1 cup honey

***

Instructions

1. Place the water and lavender in a saucepan and bring to a boil.

2. Reduce the heat and let it simmer while it is partially covered until the volume is reduced to half the original volume.

3. Strain the mixture through a sieve or cheesecloth to remove the lavender.

4. Measure 1 pint (500 mls) of the liquid and add the honey.

5. Cook for a few minutes as you stir it so that it thickens.

6. Store the syrup in an airtight container in the fridge for up to 2 months.

*****

Lavender Glycerite

Equipment

Jar with tight fitting lid

Bottle with tight fitting lid

***

Ingredients

1 cup fresh, chopped lavender or ½ cup dried, crushed lavender

2 cups vegetable glycerine

***

Instructions

1. Place the lavender in the jar and pour in the glycerine to fully cover the plant material and fill the jar.

2. Label the jar and store it in a dark place ensuring that you shake it every day.

3. After 4-6 weeks strain the lavender with a fine sieve or cheese cloth and pour the glycerite into a clean bottle.

4. Label the glycerite and store it in a cool place.

***

Tips

1. Lavender glycerites can be added to teas to sweeten and flavor them.

*****

Lavender Poultice

Equipment

Cheesecloth or old cotton sheet strips

***

Ingredients

1 tablespoon bruised fresh lavender or powdered dry lavender

Boiling water

***

Instructions

1. Add enough boiling water to the lavender to wet it and make a thick paste.

2. Spoon the lavender paste onto the cheesecloth (or bed sheet strips) to make the poultice.

3. To use, apply the poultice to the affected area and cover with another piece of hot, wet cloth. Replace the hot, wet cloth when it cools with another hot one to keep the poultice hot.

*****

Lavender Infused Oil

Equipment
Double boiler

Large glass bowl

Sieve and cheesecloth

Sterilized dark jars

***

Ingredients
16 fl oz. (500 ml) vegetable oil like organic olive, sweet almond oil or sunflower oil

8 oz. (250 grams) slightly crushed, dry lavender or 16 oz. (500 grams) slightly bruised, fresh lavender

***

Instructions
1. Place the lavender and oil in the glass bowl ensuring that the oil covers the herb. Simmer them in a double boiler for 1 hour at around 120 degrees F (49 degrees C). Do not let the mixture boil. You can repeat this step after letting the oils cool.

2. Strain the mixture through the sieve and cheesecloth into a clean, dark jar ensuring you squeeze out as much oil as you can from the cheesecloth.

3. Label your jars and store your lavender infused oils in a cool dark place or in the refrigerator and use them within 3 months.

*****

Lavender Salve

Equipment

Double boiler

Large glass bowl

Sterilized dark jars or tins

***

Ingredients

8 oz. (250 ml or 1 cup) lavender infused vegetable oil (see previous recipe)

1 oz. (30 grams) beeswax

10 drops essential oils like lavender essential oil (optional natural fragrance)

***

Instructions

1. Place the beeswax and lavender infused oil in the glass bowl and melt them in a double boiler.

2. Once melted remove from the heat source, allow to cool and add the essential oils (if using).

3. Pour the melted oils into the storage jars or tins and allow to cool completely.

4. Store the salves in a cool dark place.

*****

Lavender Lip Balm

Equipment

Double boiler

Large glass bowl

Lip balm tubes or small jars or tins

***

Ingredients

3 tablespoons lavender infused vegetable oil (see recipe above)

1 tablespoon grated beeswax

1 tablespoon shea butter

***

Instructions

1. Place the beeswax, shea butter and lavender infused oil in the glass bowl and melt them in a double boiler.

2. Once melted remove from the heat source and pour into lip balm tubes and allow to cool completely.

*****

Lavender Butter

Equipment

Large glass bowl

Electric mixer or stick blender or wire whisk

Molds such as ice cube trays (optional)

*

Ingredients

½ cup butter

2 tablespoons of finely crushed, dried lavender or 2 tablespoons of finely minced, fresh lavender

*

Instructions

1. Place the butter in a warm place so that it can soften.

2. Put butter and lavender in a large glass bowl and blend well until thoroughly mixed.

3. Refrigerate until it hardens. You can refrigerate it in molds or ice cube trays to give it a special shape.

**

Lavender Vinegar

Equipment

Large glass bottle with a well-fitting, non-metal lid or cork

***

Ingredients

2 cups white wine vinegar

1 cup lavender

***

Instructions

1. Place the lavender in the glass bottle.

2. Add the vinegar and fill the bottle to the top ensuring all the lavender is covered by vinegar.

3. Seal the bottle and let it stand for 6 weeks to 6 months. The longer it stands, the stronger the flavor becomes.

4. Strain the lavender before using the vinegar.

###

ABOUT THE AUTHOR

Marian Kim is an experienced alternative medicine practitioner.

*****

OTHER BOOKS BY THE AUTHOR

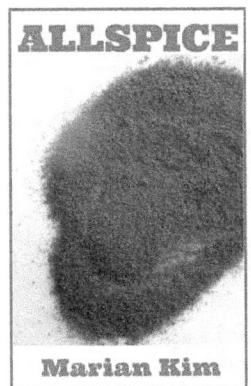

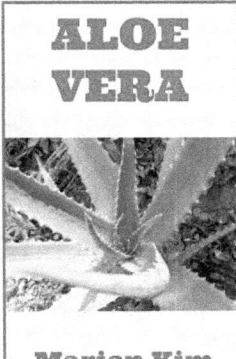

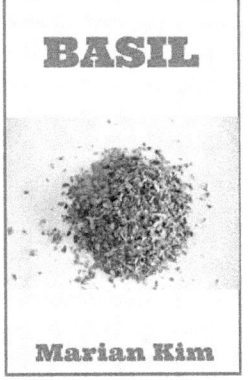

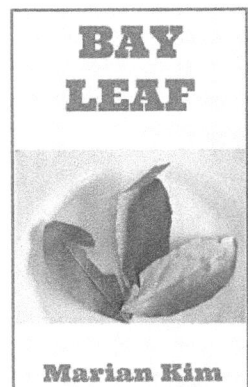

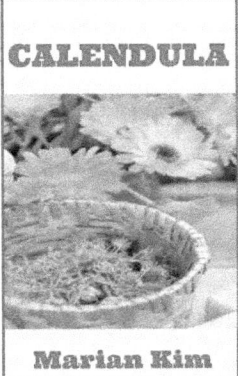

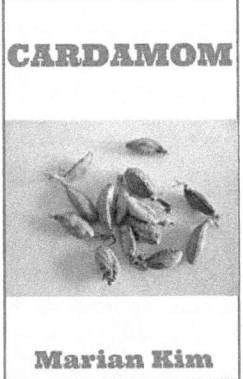

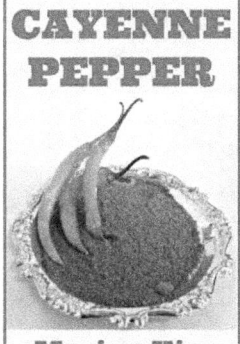
CAYENNE PEPPER
Marian Kim

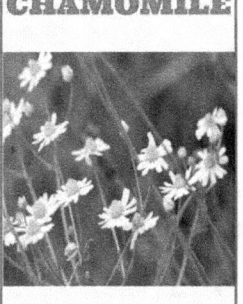
CHAMOMILE
Marian Kim

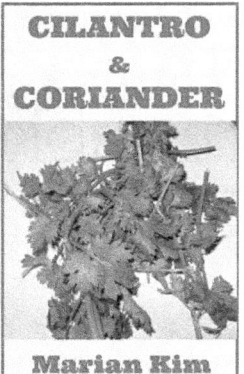
CILANTRO & CORIANDER
Marian Kim

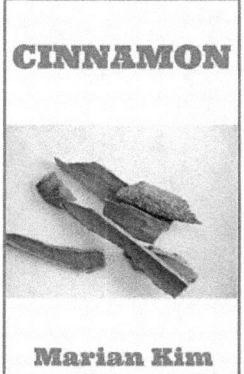
CINNAMON
Marian Kim

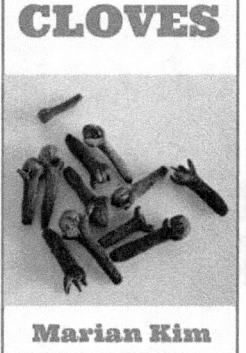
CLOVES
Marian Kim

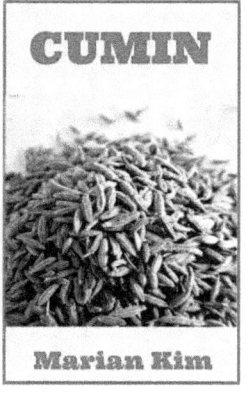
CUMIN
Marian Kim

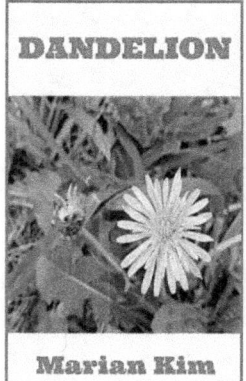
DANDELION
Marian Kim

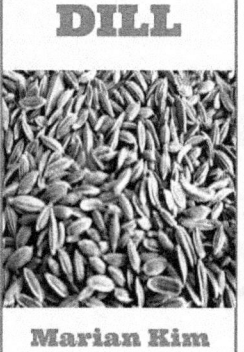
DILL
Marian Kim

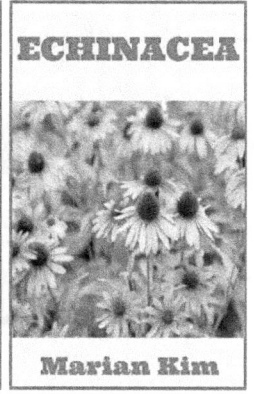
ECHINACEA
Marian Kim

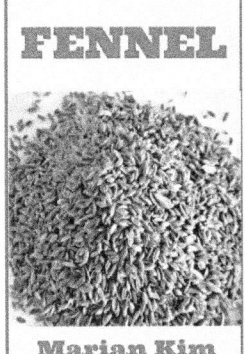

FENNEL

Marian Kim

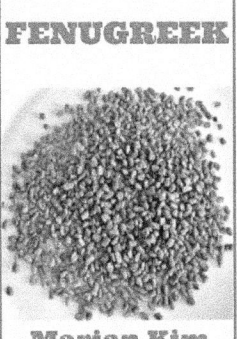

FENUGREEK

Marian Kim

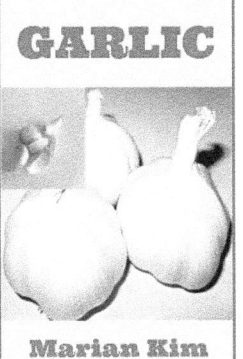

GARLIC

Marian Kim

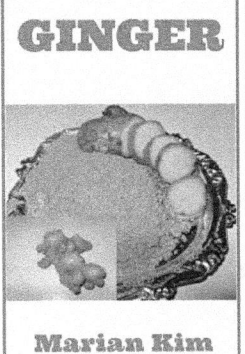

GINGER

Marian Kim

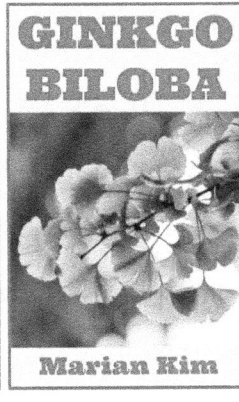

GINKGO BILOBA

Marian Kim

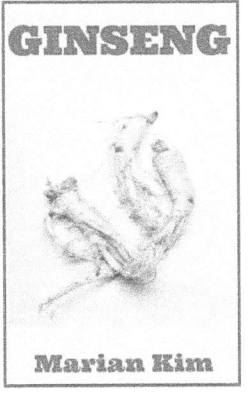

GINSENG

Marian Kim

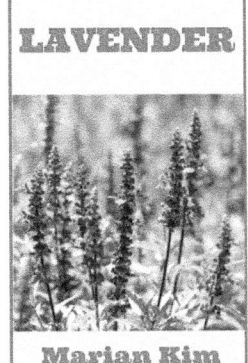

LAVENDER

Marian Kim

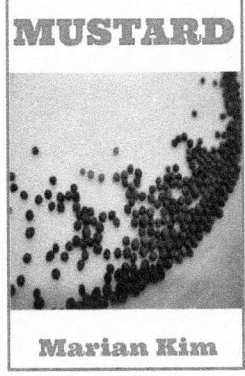

MUSTARD

Marian Kim

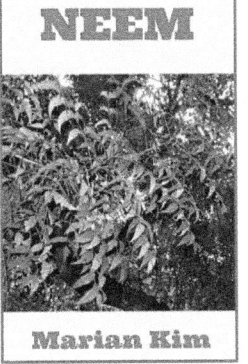

NEEM

Marian Kim

NUTMEG & MACE

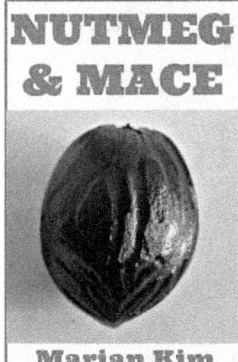

Marian Kim

OREGANO

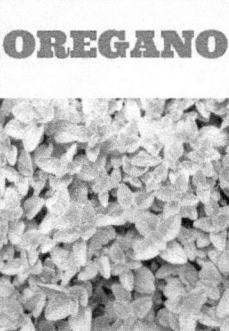

Marian Kim

PAPRIKA

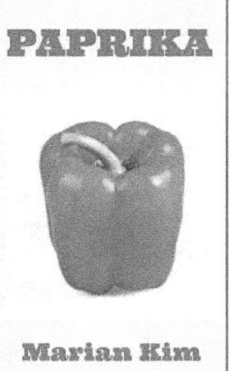

Marian Kim

PARSLEY

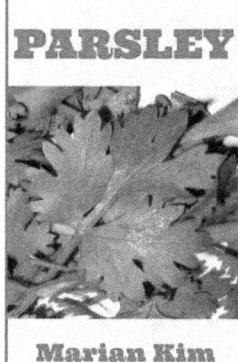

Marian Kim

BLACK & WHITE PEPPER

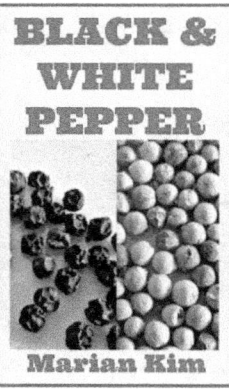

Marian Kim

PEPPERMINT

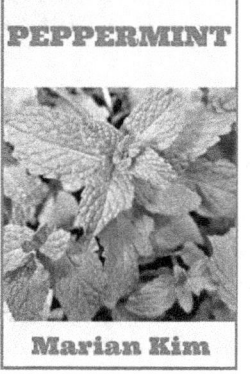

Marian Kim

ROSE HIPS

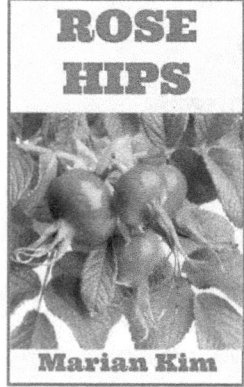

Marian Kim

ROSE PETALS

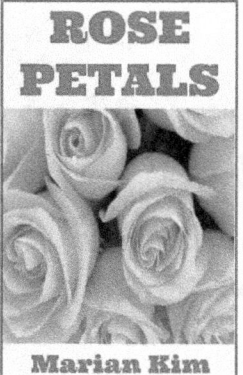

Marian Kim

ROSEMARY

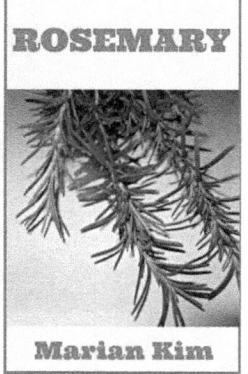

Marian Kim

SAGE

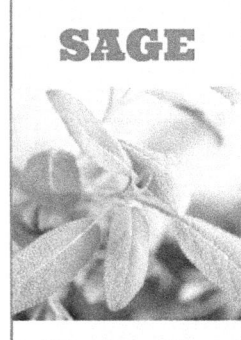

Marian Kim

ST. JOHN'S WORT

Marian Kim

STAR ANISE

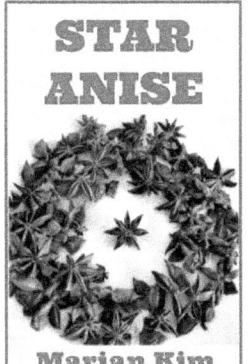

Marian Kim

STINGING NETTLE

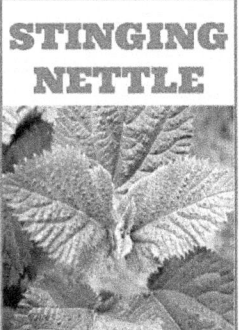

Marian Kim

THYME

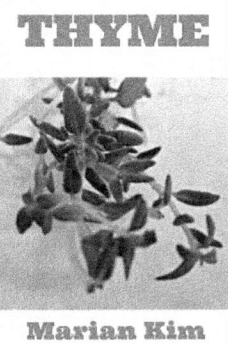

Marian Kim

TURMERIC

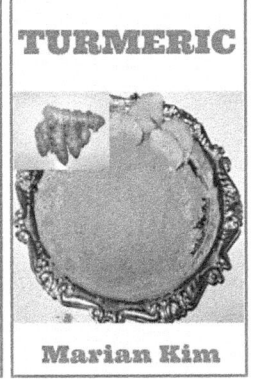

Marian Kim

WITCH HAZEL

Marian Kim

YARROW

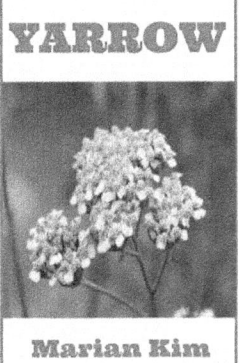

Marian Kim

*****

www.ingramcontent.com/pod-product-compliance
Lightning Source LLC
Chambersburg PA
CBHW070523290526
45790CB00003B/1273